Aging Gracefully

With Health and Dignity

Tips to Slow down the Natural Aging Process

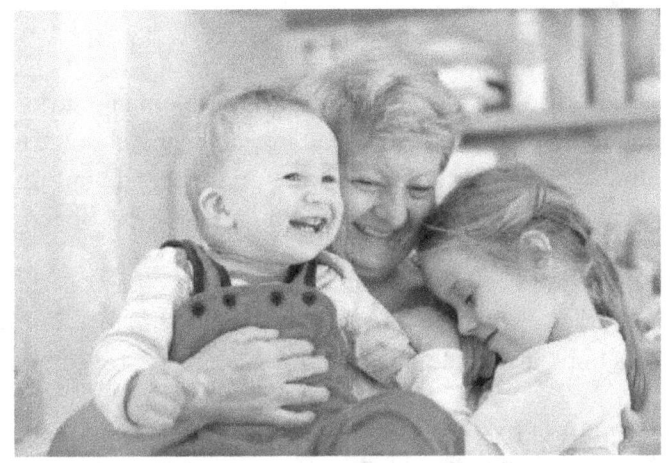

Natural Health Series

Dueep J Singh

Mendon Cottage Books

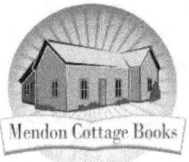

JD-Biz Publishing

Download Free Books!

http://MendonCottageBooks.com

Check out some of the other Healthy Gardening Series books at Amazon.com

Gardening Series on Amazon

Check out some of the other Health Learning Series books at Amazon.com

Health Learning Series on Amazon

Download Free Books!

http://MendonCottageBooks.com

Table of Contents

Introduction.. 4

What Is Old Age?... 6

Symptoms of Old Age.. 9

What Are the Reasons of the Natural Aging Process?........... 11

Effect of Old Age on Your Bones...................................... 13

How to Prevent Old Age Related Health Problems 16

Keeping Old Age at Bay 17

Fasting.. 20

    Rules of Fasting 20

    Knowing more about "Fasting" 22

Fruit as Cell Rejuvenators.. 28

What Do You Eat? 31

    Garlic..32

    Grapes 33

    Salt Intake 34

    Ginger...34

    Milk..35

    Yogurt 36

    Mustard Oil 37

Getting rid of Wrinkles 38

Longevity through Positive Thinking 39

Conclusion 46

Author's Bio.. 47

Publisher... 57

Introduction

Ask a number of people out there about the thing they fear the most, and many of them are going to reply – "I am rather worried about how I am going to face old age."

Believe it or not, this is one of the most prevalent of fears, affecting the subconscious psyches of a number of us. This is a natural innate reaction to one of the natural processes of a human lifecycle. Everyone knows that they are going to face old age with the passing of time. However, for a number of us, this stage of life brings with it, its own accompanying health problems, possible financial problems, and possible spiritual, emotional and physical upheaval.

As time goes by, especially when we reach our 50s and 60s, our mind starts thinking self-consciously – "we are growing old, how are we going to get through it." Unfortunately, everyone is going to go through this particular thought process sometime or the other, in the future as they grow older.

Now, this is a reaction to our body not being as energetic as it was when we were in our 30s or 40s. We expect ourselves to dance all the night, or go on 5 mile hikes, which we could do so effortlessly 10 years ago. But, what happened as the days went by? We find ourselves ready to go to bed by 11, because we do not have the energy to go out dancing and whooping it up in the city at all hours.

We find ourselves huffing and puffing after a 1 mile walk, when once we could walk for miles with impunity. Our joints ache, and we find ourselves facing other old-age related physical and mental problems.

So this book is for all those people who are facing old-age and want to know how they can stave off its more visible effects on their hearts, bodies, minds and souls, with a little bit of easy-to-use common sense tips and application.

What Is Old Age?

Old age is a state of mind. This is not a cliché. This is not an aphorism. This is not an adage. Physical manifestations like white hair, wrinkles on the skin and other outward indicators can be considered to be the harbingers of approaching old age, but people can be ever youthful, if they know their limitations brought about by old age, and still have a happy and contented mental state.

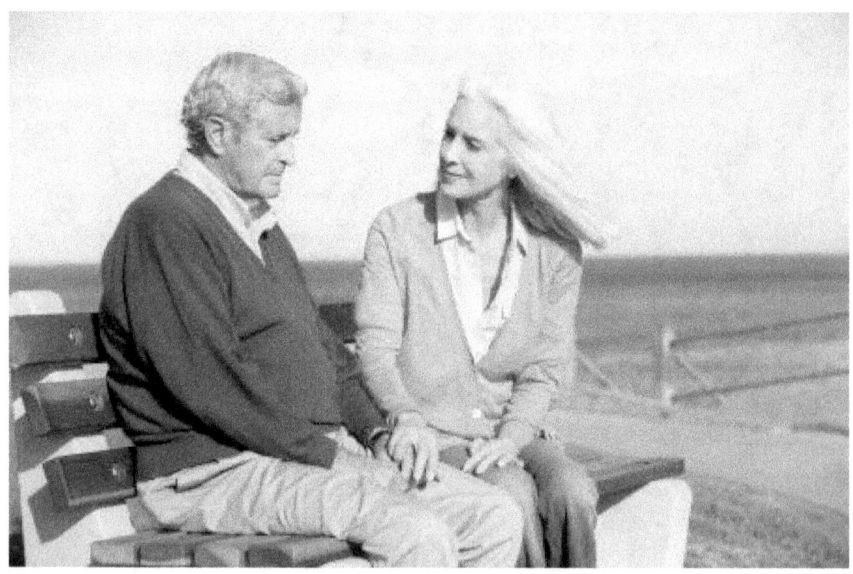

Old age is a natural stage of your life, so accept it like you accepted your childhood, youth, and middle age. Cheerful support from people of your own age group helps you to cope with this stage, especially when you feel depressed or even helpless.

In Greek mythology, they talk about the Cumaean Sibyl in those long gone days, when gods walked upon the earth seeking the love of mortals. Apollo told her that she would get whatever she desired, if she became his love. She asked for immortality, but he said that that was the prerogative of the gods and the gods alone. So she picked up a handful of sand and asked to live those many years as the grains of sand in her fist. Her wish was granted. But then Apollo, being a cunning and conniving God allowed her to live and grow old and withered until she was supposedly small enough to fit in a jar. That was because she had not asked for Eternal Youth.

Talk about unfair play. But then the ancient Greek gods are well known for their ruthlessness, especially when they are getting the better of ordinary mortals, who dared to ask them to grant mortal wishes. This 1000-year-old Sibyl supposedly dwindled away in her jar, until only her voice was left.

Down the centuries, we have found ways of prolonging lives, but we still do not know how to prevent old age. Nevertheless, growing old with dignity is the goal towards which we need to strive and this can be done only by accepting the fact that this is a natural process of life.

The only real truth in life is The Presence of Death. So this body is going to die and if you are lucky enough to have lived through a long life, and are now facing old age, you can do so with dignity.

I went to my ancestral home a couple of years ago on the death of an old and much revered relative who died at the ripe old age of 99. I was astonished to see the neighborhood preparing food and sweetmeats. In the East, it is a tradition to feed the neighborhood, the people of the town, as well as the family members with a feast, when an old wise person dies. This is a celebration of the long life he or she has led and of the heritage and legacy he or she has left behind them.

When I asked my relatives whether they were not sad that he had left us all bereft, I received the answer of "why should we be sad? He was healthy, even at 99. He was well loved by everybody in the town. He was a useful member of society. All of us took his advice, because he had the wisdom and the experience of the ages, to guide us. We miss him, but we are not going to cry because that would hold his soul from the next stage of evolution."

This is one Eastern belief, which has persisted down the ages. Apart from the part of the evolution of the soul, I was surprised at the acceptance of life-and-death. This traditional acceptance of the reality of life, and considering it in all its stages as a part of the human lifecycle is one of the reasons why the people in the East, and also in other parts of the old world, accept old age as something which has to be faced with both your eyes open. They do not begin to get tense at the onset of a couple of wrinkles or some gray hair sprinkled on their head.

And that is why they live relatively healthier and trouble-free lives, to a ripe old age.

Symptoms of Old Age

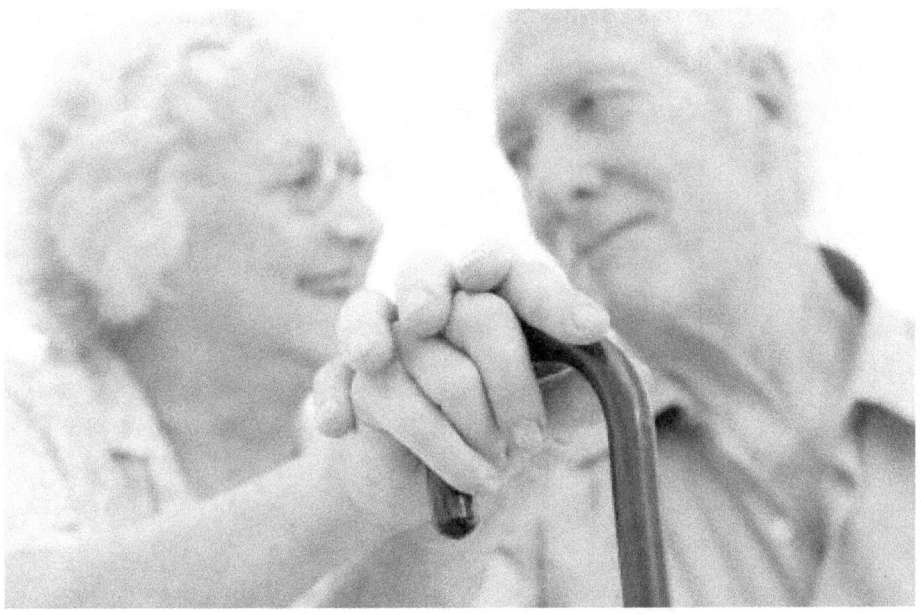

The onset of old age starts as your body starts to age. This natural aging process includes wrinkles on your skin, dry skin, weakness in your joints, stiffness in your muscles, your teeth falling out, your hair growing white, your eyes getting weaker, you needing to stoop and bend, because your spinal cord cannot support your body, incontinence, and other possible physical problems.

You cannot measure old age by years. You may see a supposedly old person more energetic than the youngsters half his age. On the other hand, there are so many youngsters out there who looked prematurely old because of their unhealthy lifestyles, bad diet, and lack of exercise. They have wrinkled skin and graying hair, even in their 30s. They may have begun to lose their teeth and they may suffer from stiff joints. So the idea that you are going to grow old, the moment you hit your 60s is not really valid or applicable, most of the time. You may also find yourself suffering from pulmonary problems like cough and colds.

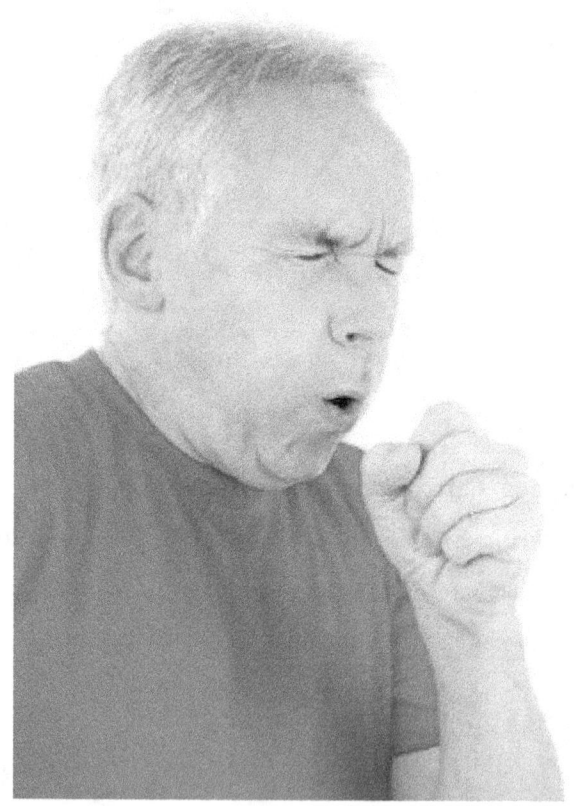

What Are the Reasons of the Natural Aging Process?

According to ancient wise men –the organs in the body slowly and steadily begin to accumulate toxic matter during the passage of time. This affects the general state of health. The rise of acidic content in the body affects the system in such a way that your gums start to swell and they may get infected, your tongue starts to tingle and its surface stays white, and other symptoms of these side effects based on this increased toxicity and acidity start to appear in your body.

This is accompanied by lethargy and the shrinking of your arteries and veins, thus lowering the efficacy of your blood circulation. Modern-day doctors are also going to give you these reasons for the natural aging process.

A cell is the unit of life, in a living body. The tissues, fibers, sinews, tendons, and each living part and organ in our bodies is made up of specialized cells which have their own particular function in the natural scheme of things. All of these living cells regenerate once every seven years, through cell division and cell regeneration continuously throughout our lifetime, thus giving rise to tissue growth and muscular growth from babyhood onwards.

The brain is also made up of nerve cells. You are going to find as many nerve cells in a normal adult's brains, as he had as a child. That is why they say that the brain keeps growing until the child is nine years old. By then 80% of the brain has developed and the rest of the development is going to be done, as he ages.

As time goes by and the body begins to age, the brain cells also start to age. Unfortunately, they do not regenerate themselves as fast as the cells found in your skin or let us say, in your bones, skin, or in other organs. Once a brain cell has been destroyed, it is not going to develop itself again through cell multiplication and division – mitosis and meiosis.

That is why, as your body ages, the cells in the brain start to dwindle away. That is the reason why people who have reached the age of 70 – 80 normally find themselves with the hearing and sight problems and have problems remembering things. That is because one fourth of these nerve cells in the brain have "died".

This is one of the side effects of old age, with the passing of time.

Effect of Old Age on Your Bones

Bone density means how many useful minerals like calcium, etc., which are normally used in the making up of bones, are present in one square inch of bone. Bone density is going to decrease as you grow older, because of the loss of calcium. This gives rise to osteoporosis. This is also the reason why so many old people start to stoop, because the bones of the spinal cord and the hip region are not strong enough to hold up the burden of the upper portion of the body.

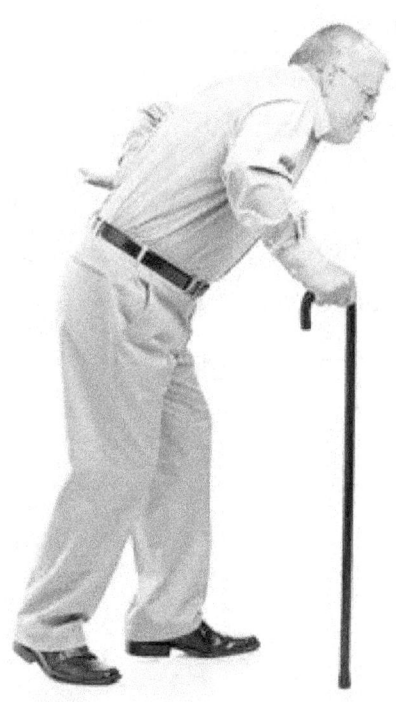

The joints of your bones are very complex in design and function. These bones are covered with a soft white layer called a cartilage and a synovial fluid presented between two joints, serves the purpose of lubricating the joint movement. With the passage of time, there is going to be a continuous "rubbing" of the joint bones, thus causing the wearing away of the cartilage. The synovial fluid is also going to lessen in quantity.

Consider an old machine with lubricating oil. Unless this oil is changed regularly for lubrication, the parts of the machine are going to grind away, until the machine breaks down. That is exactly what is going to happen to your bones, as time goes by.

This is also why we feel cramps or stiffness in our bones, when we wake up after a long night's sleep. That stiff joint and bone has not done any activity for the past eight hours. However, the moment you get up and start exercising and moving that portion of the body around, you are going to find your joints limbering up again.

As you start aging, the stiffness stays on, because the joints have grown weaker. The joints most affected are the knees, shoulders, and the backbone. You may find these portions of your body aching throughout the day.

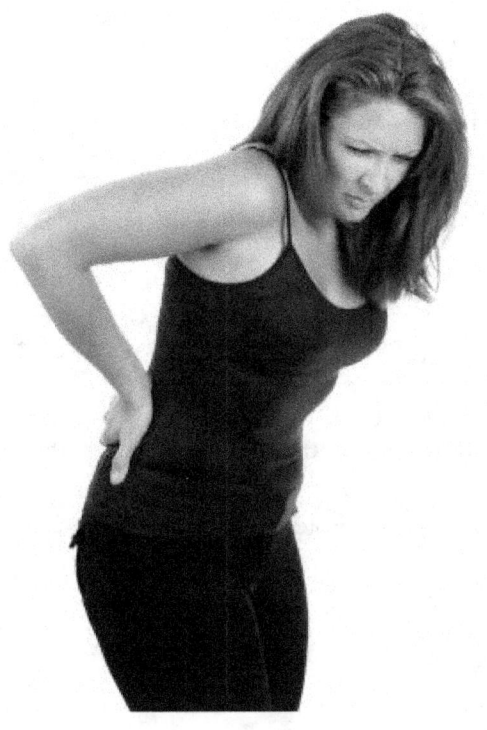

Aching joints are not restricted to just old people. They can affect anybody at any time and at any age.

How to Prevent Old Age Related Health Problems

Some of the most prevalent problems of old age include pain in the joints, lessening of vision, and feebleness. You can prevent them by eating good, balanced meals in proper healthy quantities, exercising, and preventing injury to your body.

The bones get very fragile as you grow older, so any sort of breakage in your bones is going to have a detrimental effect on your general health. That is because the bones are going to take longer to knit and heal.

These bones are made up of protein and calcium. So your diet should be full of protein and calcium-based items which are easily digested.

The average age span of a person in olden days, when there was peace, and plenty of healthy food to go around, was more than 100 years. As old as Methuselah is the well-known saying, and at that time, a long old age was a rule instead of being an exception.

However, as time went by, mankind found that it had followed in the golden rules, with which it could stay healthy and happy for a longer period of time. We are slowly and steadily learning that knowledge again, but even so, as long as we do not change our lifestyle and get back to a more natural atmosphere, we are still going to have an average lifespan of three score and ten with luck.

Believe it or not, if a person reaches the age of seventy, without succumbing to illnesses and ailments, the chances of his making it to a longer stretch of living increase proportionately.

Keeping Old Age at Bay

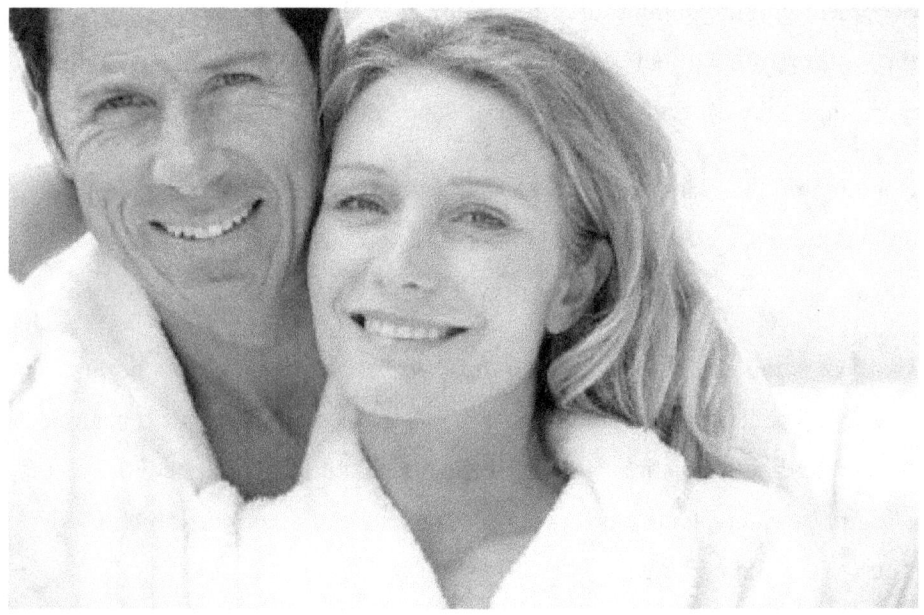

A healthy mental attitude and a cheerful and positive mental outlook towards life and the future, does much in keeping old age at bay.

In olden times, the ancients believed in four stages of life for every man. Childhood, youth and adult age was spent in gaining of knowledge, and living a householders life, raising a family and children. At the age of sixty-five, they gave up everything and retired to live a hermit's life in Hermitages, till death took them.

This stage of life was the renunciation of every material thing, and an acceptance of every spiritual thing, which gave the soul, body and heart, plenty of peace and tranquility. They used to get food and water that was given to them by the people living in the hermitages. All their old age related illnesses were treated by wise men and doctors. They would spend their time in busy physical work, when it was possible, and kept their minds occupied with the gaining of knowledge. They did not allow the problems of the world to touch them, because they were preparing themselves for the next stage of evolution – the facing of death and what came after it.

Renouncing the world and turning your back to it meant no more tension and no more worries. However, that is not so today. Everybody wants to stay as they say "in harness", along with family and its related tensions.

Here are some golden rules, which these ancients followed, millenniums ago. They kept physically active as long as they could. They ate a healthy digestible diet, consisting of fruits, vegetables, meat in small quantities, lots of dairy products, lentils and cereals and beans and other nutritional food. They never skipped meals.

They woke up at dawn and started the day's work in the fresh air and fresh new sunshine. They never felt physically exhausted because they were so used to physical labor, that the body had accustomed itself to a regular work routine, since childhood and youth. That regime persisted until the day they died.

During this time, death was normally due to accidents, war, and disease. Barring these catastrophes, the majority of people lived for a long time, and died in their beds in due course.

They kept their digestive systems active by not overloading it with lots of food. They relished the food they ate and spent some time over its eating. Here is an ancient exercise, which was done in the East, to improve the digestive system.

Lie down on your back, and lean your head forward. This is to tighten the muscles of your stomach. Now throw your head back, in the same lying down position, so that the muscles of the stomach are loosened. Keep doing this, ten times in one exercise routine. While you are doing this, raising and lowering of your head, keep punching the stomach area slowly with a closed fist.

You should start by massaging and punching that stomach area gently in the beginning, and then a little harder, after a while. This improves the circulation of the blood in the stomach area. This is also going to strengthen your digestive system. After that, massage your stomach area with the palms of your hand. This pummeling also helps in the breakage of the cellulite muscles accumulated in that particular region.

To prevent the formation of calcium in your bones with the passing of time, keep them supple by exercising them regularly. Regular walking, getting up and down the stairs, getting up from a bed or chair and then just pottering around the house keeps your joints from stiffening and lessens the chances of calcium accumulation in them.

Fasting

Fasting is a way of life in the East. Once upon a time, fasting was considered to be a part of life, because there was not enough of food to go around. That is why people had to go hungry often. This is how they found out that it was a healthy thing to have at least one hungry day in fifteen days, when people fasted.

This got rid of all the toxins in the body. Fasting meant not eating any cereals or any grain-based foods or cooked items. Water, fresh fruit and vegetables were eaten and drunk throughout the day.

Soon fasting became a way of life and it also became a religious tradition. In the Indian subcontinent, twice a year, the Hindus go through Nine days of fasting. All over the world, the Mussulmen's fast throughout one holy month and the Christians also have their own tradition of strict fasting and abstinence, especially during Lent. Other religions also know all about the importance of fasting, and follow it strictly and diligently at given periods of time.

So, apart from the spiritual benefits accrued from such abstinence, what is the physical benefit of fasting? You are ridding your body of all the toxins. You are eating healthy food items which are not a normal part of your daily diet. This change of diet helps in "tuning up" your body with more and different minerals and nutrients.

Rules of Fasting

Never starve your body completely. Fasting does not mean not eating anything at all. Staying hungry because you do not have access to food is not fasting, it is starvation. Fasting is something you do on your own accord, knowing that you have access to food whenever your body needs it.

Do not fast continuously. Your body cannot accommodate itself to sporadic periods of missed meals, all in the name of fasting. It is plenty of nutrients, minerals and other natural ingredients in order to keep functioning properly. So remember to take fruit, water, and milk at regular intervals during your fast.

You may want to take some lemon juice in water and sip it slowly throughout the day.

Your body should not get dehydrated during a fasting. That is why you need to increase your liquid intake. Fresh fruit juices are excellent to get rid of all those toxins.

In ancient times, one day in a week, was given to fasting, when a simple fruit and water diet was just what a person ate. That cleared his system of the accumulated toxins gathered in the last six days.

You do not have to have a specialized diet, when you are trying to keep old age at bay, but you would want to increase the amount of raw fruit and vegetables in your diet, along with cooked food.

It has been proved through scientific research that spices, vegetables, fruit, dry fruit, milk products, and other natural products are a treasure house of natural minerals, vitamins, fats, carbohydrates, and other natural essential nutrients necessary to keep your body healthy and fit. But, all this knowledge was known to people of ancient civilizations, ever since the dawn of mankind.

When man decided to use his brain to take notice of his surroundings, he noticed that some fruit and vegetables were good additions to his meal of hunted meat and nuts. With the passing of time, he began to use spices and herbs with his meals.

But how many of these items can an old person digest properly? Not many. That is why you may need to limit yourself to the consumption of dry fruit and spices when you are old.

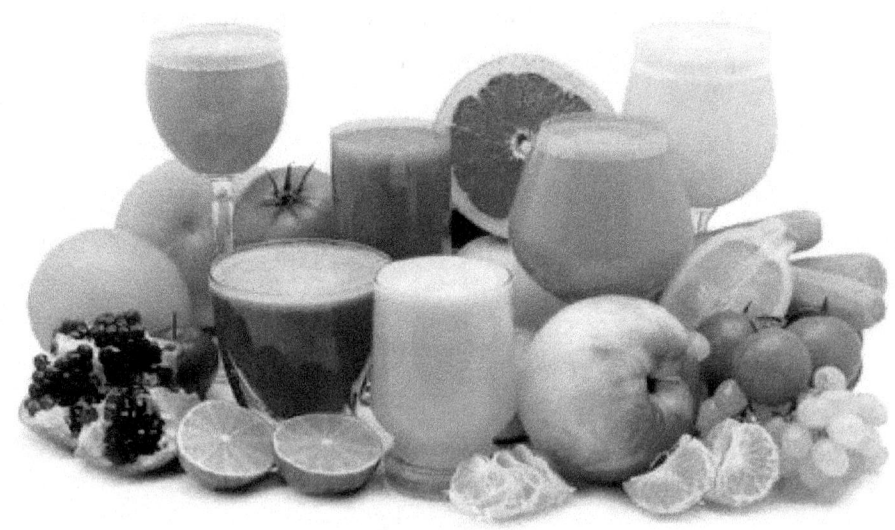

Knowing more about "Fasting"

Is it sensible for old people to "fast?"

I have noticed that as people grow older, they begin to be more "spiritual" in their outlook, and along with prayers, they begin to "fast" even more. A fast means the total abstinence from eating any kind of food. That means you are not going to take any liquid or solid food, fruit, cereals and water. This is done for a definite period, with a view of giving rest to the different organs of the body, and detoxifying it. This is also supposed to be a purification of the mind, spirit and body.

Is this fasting a healthy activity, you may ask? Well, I can clearly say that this definitely is not advisable for old people, from keeping healthy point of view, even though conventional traditionalists, used to fasting, will not agree with me. That is because in plenty of societies all over the world, fasting, at regular periods is a way of life. But then, this does not include eating and drinking *absolutely nothing at all* throughout the day.

Since ancient times, man has been fasting for a number of reasons – both practical and religious. That is why he normally abstained from eating food on a particular day. In olden times, it had nothing to do with religion, but had more to do with whether the hunter of the tribe managed to get a good catch during the day. If he could not manage to catch anything, the people of the tribe just drank some water, and went off to sleep hungry. This is not "fasting." This is reality brought on by circumstances.

As time went by, people began to abstain from food as a matter of a religious practice, considering it to be a way to achieve some spiritual state of well-being. Priests abstained from food at one meal time or even one day, before the celebration of some holy festival.

This sort of detoxification for just about 8 – 10 hours is acceptable, because your body is not being starved. Remember that your body needs lots of minerals, proteins, carbohydrates, and other essential nutrients in order to function properly. People above the age of 60 cannot afford any sort of malnutrition. They also cannot afford to starve their bodies of these essential nutrients.

However, if they intend to fast – putting aside any religious significance – the fasting can be done by taking fruit, water or fruit juices. At least the stomach is getting some sort of nutrient and there is no chance of its missing out on liquid intake, which is necessary to keep your body healthy and strong.

Fasting does not mean starving like I said. Fasting and starving are 2 different conditions. It is true that in both these conditions, you do not eat anything. But fasting is done voluntarily. Starving is either done due to force of circumstances when you do not have food to eat, or possibly when you are so sick that you cannot manage to eat any food. That means that you are going to suffer from starvation in the long run.

Starving is beyond the control of an individual. When you are sick, your body is going to be using all its power in order to counteract the disease and help heal your body naturally. During this period, your body requires more nourishment, but because it is not functioning normally, you may not feel hungry. But remember that the regular elimination of toxins accumulating in your body needs to take place, whether you are healthy or when you are sick.

When your body does not need any nourishment, and your appetite is dormant, any sort of abstention from eating can be considered to be fasting. Remember that your body requires heat and fuel, even while you are fasting. That is when your body begins to burn all the "fuel", already present in it to keep it functioning normally, because it knows that it is not going to have food coming in soon.

Starvation is going to be the condition in which your cells and organs are slowly going to deteriorate because of continuous fasting. If you have been fasting over a long period of time, you are going to find yourself starving and suffering from malnutrition.

Fasting in order to lose weight is the new 21st-century fad. This is why many people suffer from eating disorders. They are depriving their body of the essential natural nutrients required to keep healthy. They may lose weight temporarily, but that is because the body has rid itself of the accumulated toxins. But all that weight is going to come back again, as soon as they start eating again.

An old person cannot afford to have the essential stored fuel in his body "burned" up, because he is not eating. This burning process includes the catabolism of fat and blood sugar. If the fastest continued after all the present body fat is used up, the fibers and the cells of your organs are going to disintegrate and a desperate body is going to derive its nourishment from them. This is definitely harmful and potentially dangerous.

A majority of people nowadays "fast" for anywhere between 9 to 10 days to one month, for a number of reasons, including possible spiritual progress and mental peace. But this fasting process does not mean that they deprive their body of essential nutrients. The body is fed fruit juices, fresh fruit, and other fast related foods, which means that the system is still working in a healthy fashion, even though the diet has changed.

Simple, light and nutritious food should be taken for the period of the fast. Raw vegetables, sprouted cereals, and sprouted pulses should be taken in large quantities so that your body is not deprived of minerals and vitamins needed to detoxify it.

In addition to this, the surplus vitamins and nutrients are stored away in the body, to be used at will, if the person is determined to extend his fasting period.

At the time of ending the fast, you need to end it with a little quantity of orange juice or lemon juice. That is because the digestive system has been comparatively inactive during this period. The intestines may have shrunk in size, if the fasting was done over a longer period of time. Great care needs to be taken before burdening these "dormant" digestive organs, with a heavy meal. For the first couple of days, drink just fruit juices. After 4 – 5 days, you can take boiled vegetables and cooked food should be given after a week or so.

Old people should never be allowed to fast, because any sort of abstinence from meals is going to have a detrimental effect on their naturally weakening bodies. If they persist on fasting, feed them plenty of fruit and vegetables. Make sure that they have some sort of cooked food at least once a day. This is going to prevent their intestines from "shrinking".

Giving them lots of rich and fatty food in the hope that they are going to regain their energy and weight lost during a fast is dangerous and foolish.

Remember that the necessity of fasting is going to arise only when you have not bothered much about regular meals, proper diet, and proportion of diet when you eat and drink. You can go through a lifetime without fasting, if you have followed "proper eating" rules throughout your life.

The fasting process is done to detoxify your body. The moment you start eating a rich diet again after a fast, your body is going to become a storehouse of these poisonous elements and toxins which cause diseases, yet once again. You can miss a meal once a week, if you have been eating regular meals 3 times a day throughout your life. But missing meals regularly, and thinking that you are fasting, and you are thus losing weight is misleading. You are just harming your body.

Fruit as Cell Rejuvenators

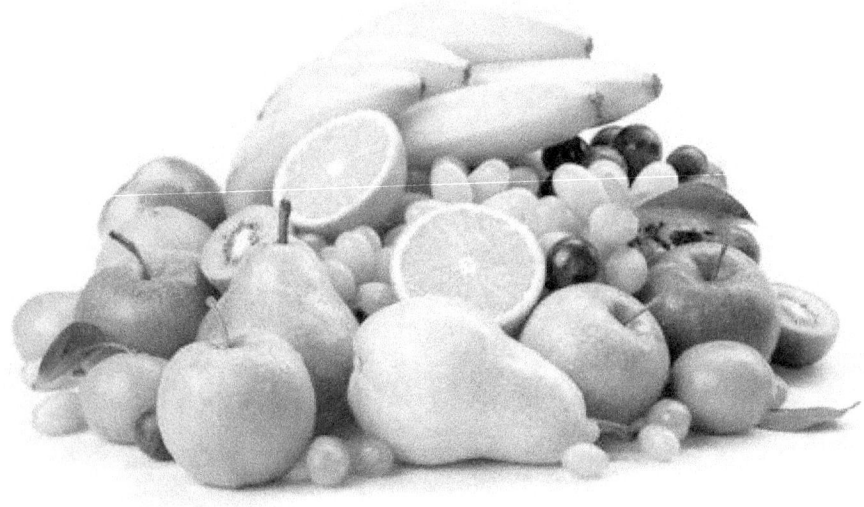

Did you know that fruit are just one of the most important natural products, which help in the growth of new cells, and rejuvenating them in your body? When you are getting ready for your old age, try this diet regime of just a strict fruit diet for a month, at least once a year. Eat the seasonal fruits present in that particular season for that whole month. This not only gives you plenty of body resistance, but it also helps you maintain body strength.

Fruit reduce the acidity level in your body, and gets rid of the toxins. They also help improve the immunity system of your body.

It does not depend on what you eat, which is going to improve your health, but it is going to depend on what you digest, which is going to make all the difference between a healthy body and an ailing body. So, a healthy digestive system, assimilating food which can be easily digested is going to be much better for an aging body.

Remember to eat food whenever you feel hungry. Most of us have this bad habit of grabbing the latest edible item in front of us, whenever we want, or if we are feeling bored, or if we are watching a movie, or we are doing something and want to accompany that action with something on which to chew.

This tendency is the reason why so many of us suffer from obesity, as well as eating disorders. That is because we eat everything and anything indiscriminately and at all hours. This is not a thing which you should follow in your 20s, 30s and 40s. In your childhood and adolescent years, you need to eat lots of food, in order to grow in a healthy manner. But, if you continue this practice, when you are a full-grown adult, you are only going to gain weight.

Rich meals are not going to give you plenty of nutrition, even though they are tasty. Also, do not overeat. I have found a really good way to enjoy my food, especially when I want to eat something and I am scared that the calories are going to count against my weight loss diet program.

Smaller portions of meals, and even smaller helpings can give your stomach plenty of nutrition. Try it this experiment today. Overfill your plate with lots of food. What is your first reaction? Oh my, I need to eat all this. And you begin to do that. There you are, you have overeaten, beyond what your body needed.

The second part of the experiment is going to be done on your next meal. Take smaller helpings. Half of the amount that you took in your last meal is going to do you just fine. Your first reaction is – I will still stay hungry, if I eat so little. The answer to this reaction is, oh, I need not worry, I can come back and take another helping, if I want to.

It has been scientifically proven that this mental autosuggestion makes you finish everything which is in your plate and most often, unless you intend to finish one particular tasty dish in one particular sitting, you do not go back for second helpings.

Your digestive power and diet capacity when you grow old is going to be diminished. So this is the only time when you are going to eat, at all hours of the day, eat small amounts of food, enough to nourish you and to keep you healthy. Do not overeat.

What Do You Eat?

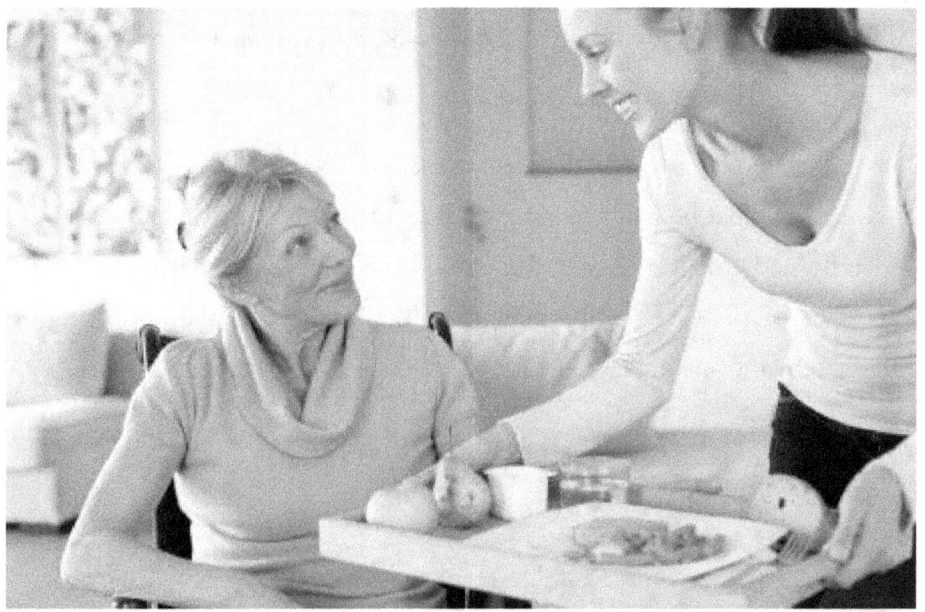

Light food, in small quantities can help keep the elderly healthy and well fed.

After you have done the morning exercise, you may want to break your fast on the diet of the ancients. This was made up of milk, without any sugar, three bananas, four dates and a little bit of coconut, if you can manage to chew it. The coconut was to "oil" the body and clear the system. The dates were to give you energy and manufacture more blood. Dates also prevented incontinence, especially in older people.

The combination of milk and bananas has been considered to be the best complete food combination down the ages.

In the afternoon, you would want to eat 60 g of whole wheat bread, rice, seasonal vegetables, both cooked and uncooked. Sugarcane juice is very healthy, so drink it when you can.

In the evening, you are going to drink milk, and seasonal fruit, along with some dry fruit.

I asked a person, who was in his 90s, the secret of his longevity. He answered me that he had a healthy breakfast and a healthy lunch, but he had just milk and fruit for dinner. He started this diet when in his 40s, and it persisted for the next half a century. I believe this was the diet regime followed by the ancients.

Garlic

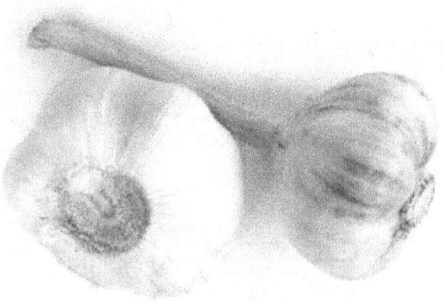

Along with that, they ate plenty of garlic in their diet. This slowed down the natural aging process considerably.

Mix one part of crushed garlic with four parts of honey. Take 2 teaspoons of this mixture twice a day. 50 days are enough to tune up your immunity system, get rid of infections, and fill you up with lots of energy and vigor. Garlic is an herb which is a magic rejuvenator. If you don't want to take the trouble of doing this, you can chew 4 cloves of raw garlic, with a glassful of water or boil it in a glassful of water at least once a day.

Add 2 cloves of raw garlic to your lunch, right now.

Grapes

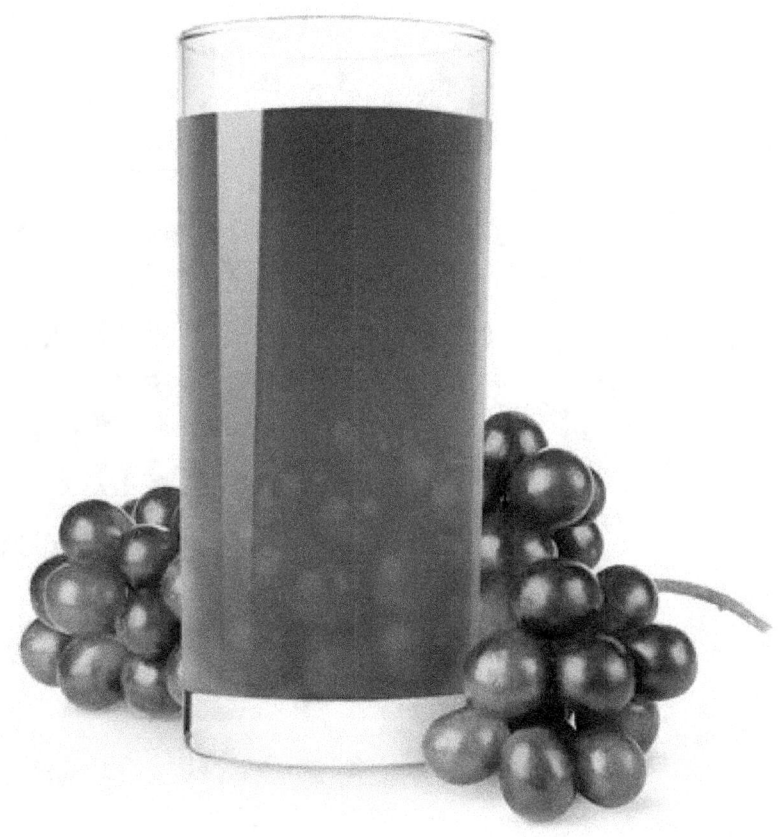

Grapes are essential to keep you healthy fit and fine. Raisins need to be eaten by old people every day because they provide you with immunity to diseases as well as help in the manufacture of blood. The sugar provided by the grapes and raisins are easily digested and assimilated by your body.

Salt Intake

In the olden days, old people were not given salt to eat, because it was said that salt brought about the onset of old age. The food was spiced with herbs and spices in such a manner that they did not feel the absence of salt. You may also want to try to reduce your salt intake in your diet from now onwards.

Ginger

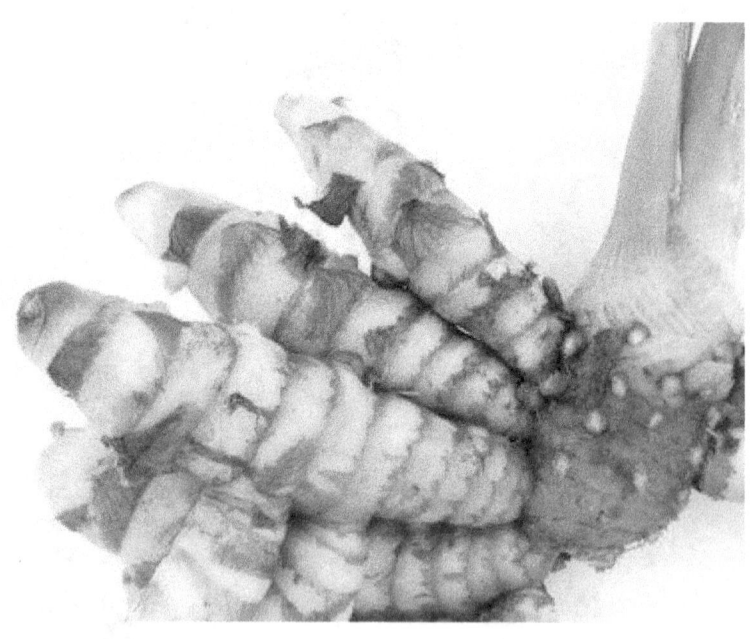

Ginger not only gingers up your system, but it is one of the healthiest herbs known to mankind. Remember to eat a bean sized piece of ginger, 15 minutes before you eat a meal. This is going to keep your digestive system healthy. It is also going to improve your immune system.

Milk

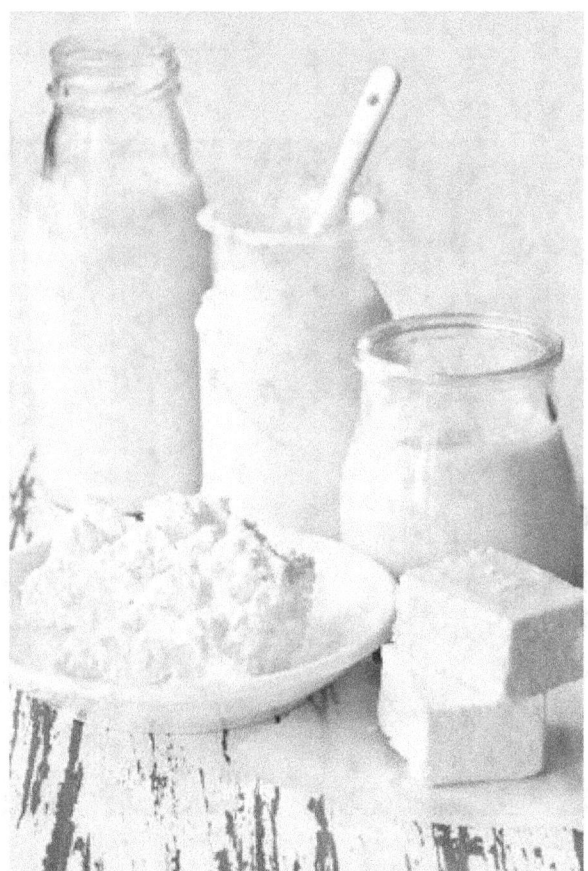

Milk has been an important part of the human diet for millenniums, so it is surprising why adults have stopped drinking it regularly. Instead, they poison their system with caffeine and Tea. Try drinking milk with your lunch. In the Indian subcontinent, milk is given to adults with 3 teaspoons full of honey and one teaspoonful of clarified butter – known as desi ghee.

As people in the West do not believe in eating fat, because of their sedentary lifestyle, I would suggest drinking milk and honey instead. After all, it has been praised by Wise men down the ages!

Yogurt

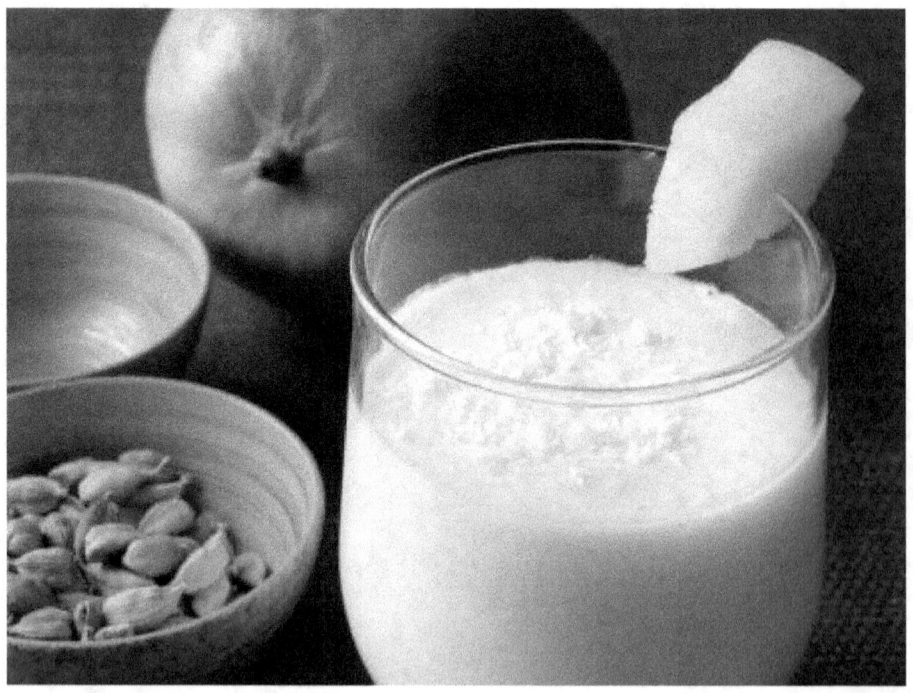

Yogurt needs to be a part of your daily diet in some form or the other. So remember to take it with your lunch or dinner. You can also drink buttermilk

Mustard Oil

He gave me another tip- when he was in his 40's, he began putting two drops of mustard oil in his ears before he went off to sleep. According to him, this was what kept old age, at bay for a long while, and also kept his hearing, and vision, as well as his teeth healthy.

In Europe, especially in Greece and Spain, old people are massaged with olive oil. This is an ancient tradition. In the East, they are massaged with coconut oil and mustard oil, and then allowed to bask in the sun. This keeps their limbs in good condition and supple.

Getting rid of Wrinkles

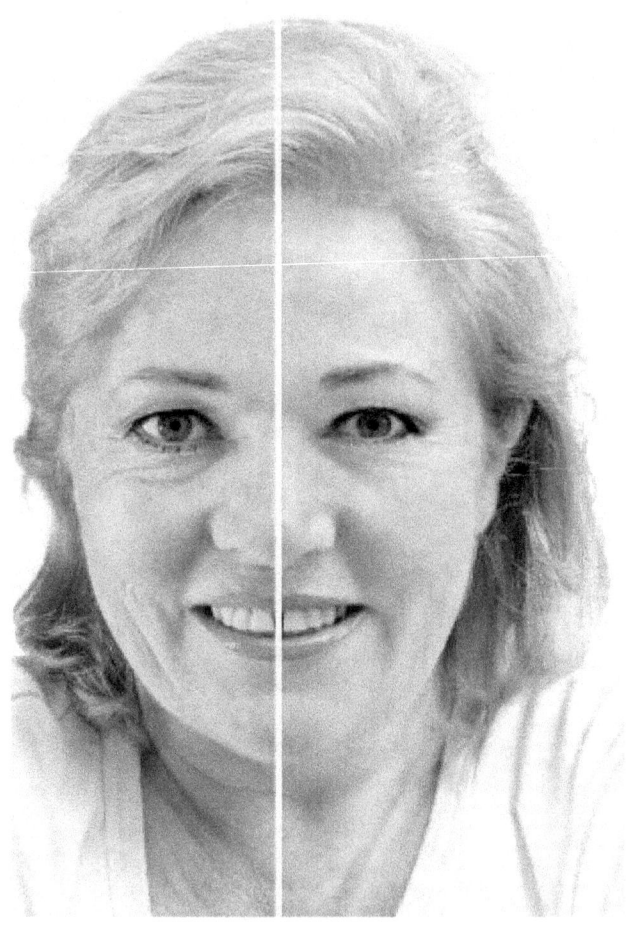

I know of a relative in her 80s who has a beautifully smooth unwrinkled face. Her secret is that since her 40s, she added honey to lemon juice, and massaged her face and neck with this mixture. It kept her skin moisturized. Wrinkles never formed. So if you have wrinkles on your face, you may want to get rid of them, with this excellent natural wrinkle remover.

Longevity through Positive Thinking

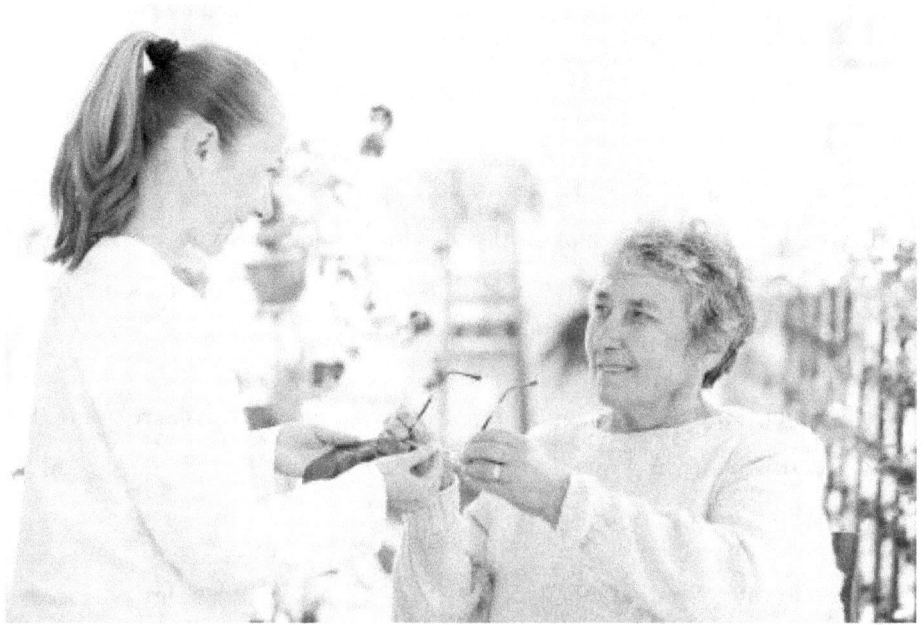

Nowadays, we may say that we do not have the time to do all these little caring things for old people, but that just shows how callous and careless we are growing towards people who are approaching the sunset of their lives.

We just put them in nursing homes, and put our responsibility towards them in the hands of medical professionals and caretakers. Unfortunately, this attitude is spreading all over the world, and is one of the reasons why many people fear the advent of old age. In ancient times, they never had to fear growing old and being neglected by the people of their village, family, or tribe.

They tell a very thought-provoking story about a family, where grandpa was being taken care of by his son and daughter-in-law. The young grandson soon found out that his grandfather was being neglected by his parents. They didn't bother much about giving him food and drink at regular times. Grandpa did not dare protest, because there was nowhere else for him to go and no one else to care for him.

One day the grandson saw that his grandfather was being fed bread and meat on a wooden platter. That supposedly was good enough for the old man of the house. The next day the father saw his son whittling away on a piece of wood. "What are you doing my boy?" he asked.

"Well, father, I am just making a platter for you, on which you are going to be fed food, when you grow old. When I finish making this platter, I need to make another one for mother. "

Needless to say, grandfather was treated like a king from that day onwards till the day he died.

So, if we understand the fact, that old age is the stage when the older generation needs our loving care, support and also the feeling that they are needed and they are wanted, the willpower to live is going to remain strong.

Your willpower has a direct effect on your health. The moment a person feels the onset of old age, he begins to think that he has reached a stage when he is of no use to anyone. But willpower is going to keep this idea out of your mind. This idea is very detrimental to your psyche, your emotional well-being, your spiritual and mental health, as well as, your physical strength and health.

The feeling of stress and strain, brought about by a mental tension of "I am getting old, I am going to be powerless to do this particular activity, or work – be it physical or mental –" is one of the reasons why people find their physical and mental health going downhill fast.

That is because they have auto – suggested themselves into a state, when they think that as they are old, they are a possibly useless and neglected quantity in the social fabric.

This mental attitude was not present in society millenniums ago. Old people were revered. They were looked up to, as they were considered to be the teachers of the younger generation. They were taken care of well and it was considered to be a privilege to take care of them, all the while gaining benefit of their knowledge as well as also gaining good "karma."

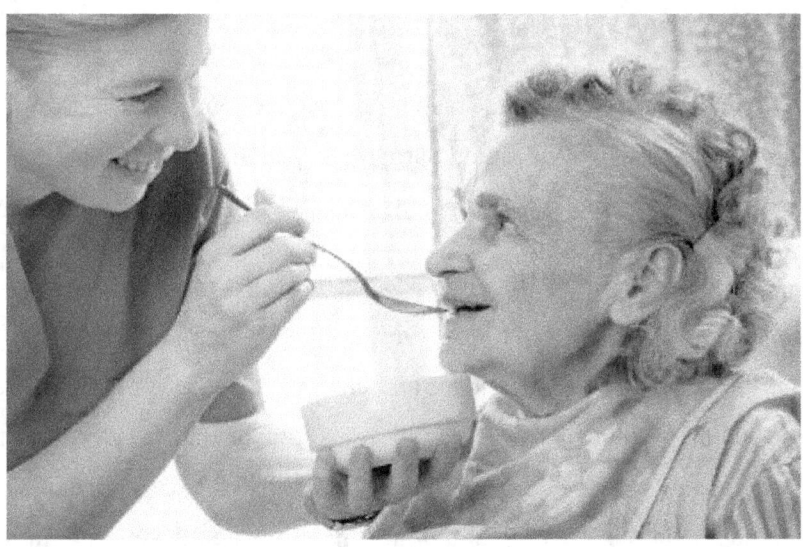

The old not only need physical care, but they also need the personalized human touch, which should be sincere and patient.

That sort of feeling is quite rare nowadays, because has become more self-centered and selfish. He could not be bothered to take care of an old person in the family. Instead, he tries his best to make that old person feel mentally and spiritually diminished by saying "father, you are growing old, and you really do not know what you are saying."

I would not be surprised if you have heard the same words being spoken by people of your acquaintance, to their elders, in a tone of patronizing superiority and contempt.

2000 years ago, an old father could punish his son for daring to say these words to him, even though the son was the head of his own household, in his own right. But today, a father better not remonstrate with his son, because you never know, the son may just lift up his hand and knock his old father about, because, hey, he is a man. [Unfortunately, I have seen scenes of such domestic violence against old people being done by negligent caretakers as well as by members of the family.]

This is a matter of global social shame. And we call ourselves civilized. In fact, those ancient tribes we called barbarians, pagans and heathens millenniums ago were more civilized than us, because they revered their old people and treated them with respect.

So remember, there is a time when you are also going to grow old. If you are lucky enough to be independent and can take care of yourself, well, you are fortunate. On the other hand, there is the chance that your family members may decide to fob off their responsibility of taking care of you on the shoulders of the government or the national healthcare programs for seniors. Once they have done that, they think it enough to visit you once every six months, for about half an hour taken from their busy schedule.

And then they go out and talk to the doctor, "what is the matter with my father, Doctor? I can see that his condition is worsening. His state of mind and physical health is deteriorating fast. I am paying you enough to take care of him, so why are you not doing that?"

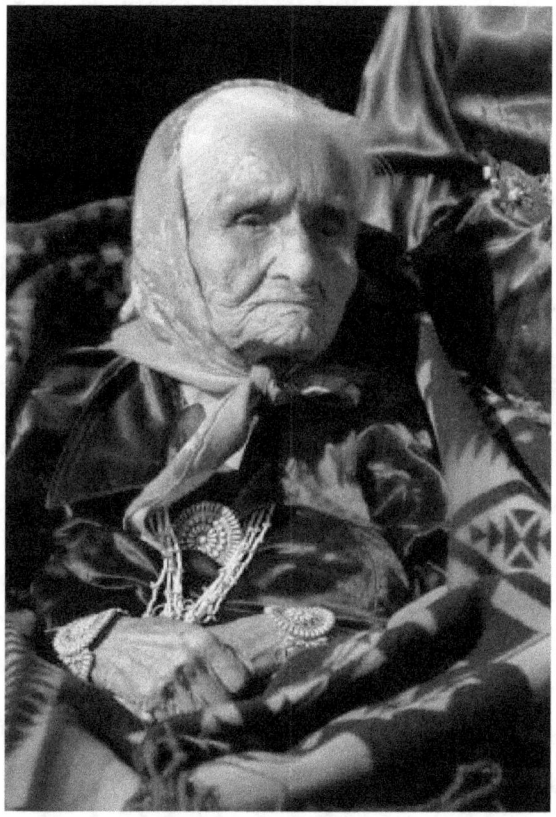

Growing old with pride and dignity is one's Birthright.

Notice something here? This conscientious son is making it clear that he is worried about the state of his father's health, based on a one hour visit every six months or so. He has not bothered to find out about the emotional state of a parent, left with doctors and caretakers who definitely do not take the part of family, nor can they give an old person, the personalized affection, care and support he needs.

He also does not hesitate to chastise the doctor about not taking care of his father, because that is the only way in which he can assuage his guilt – if he feels any – with a reassurance that his job is done for another six months.

Many children think that paying others to take care of their parents is quite enough, because they really cannot take the time to do so themselves. The state of irresponsibility, unfortunately, is becoming the rule, instead of the exception, in the 21st century, where the sunset and twilight of many lives are spent in cold, sterile, and warmth free old age homes and hospitals.

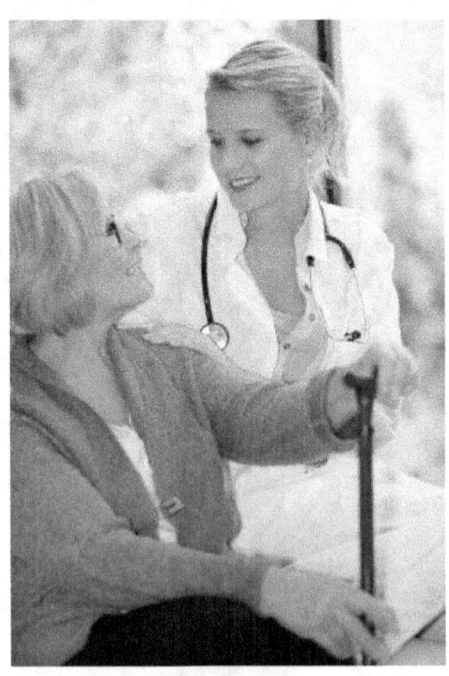

So looking forward to such a state, especially for you, is definitely not something on which people wish to dwell. But, this is a natural way of life, in most parts of the world in the 21st century. Governments may start up programs for the care of their older citizens, but they still have a long way to go in treating them as valuable, useful, and still wanted and needed people in their own rights.

Conclusion

I was reading a book about The Second World War, telling the story of a Navy officer who was unable to join up on the outset of the war. He was supposedly too old.

His daughter-in-law soon noticed that her father-in-law had not only given up sugar, but he had also given up eggs, bread, milk and other then available food items, because he considered himself a useless mouth. He had slowly begun to starve himself, because nobody wanted him.

Luckily, she was sensible enough to get in touch with the Ministry of Defense and tell them about taking full advantage of an experienced admiral, who considered himself of no use to the King and Country. That was because he had asked to join up and some rude and harassed person had told him in no uncertain terms that they really could not be bothered with old fogeys.

The minister was intelligent and sensible, and sent an official car to collect the Admiral the very next morning because his country needed him. Needless to say, the Admiral got a new lease of life and served his country well throughout the war, in strategy planning and administration.

Remember, old age is a state of mind and stage of life when people get depressed, because they are not physically and mentally strong. So they need all your support, love, care, and affection. So allow and help them to grow old with dignity and grace, because one day you will be in their shoes.

Author's Bio

Dueep Jyot Singh is a Management and IT Professional who managed to gather Postgraduate qualifications in Management and English and Degrees in Science, French and Education while pursuing different enjoyable career options like being an hospital administrator, IT,SEO and HRD Database Manager/ trainer, movie , radio and TV scriptwriter, theatre artiste and public speaker, lecturer in French, Marketing and Advertising, ex-Editor of Hearts On Fire (now known as Solstice) Books Missouri USA, advice columnist and cartoonist, publisher and Aviation School trainer, ex-moderator on Medico.in, banker, student councilor ,travelogue writer … among other things!

One fine morning, she decided that she had enough of killing herself by Degrees and went back to her first love -- writing. It's more enjoyable! She already has 48 published academic and 14 fiction- in- different- genre books under her belt.

When she is not designing websites or making Graphic design illustrations for clients , she is browsing through old bookshops hunting for treasures, of which she has an enviable collection – including R.L. Stevenson, O.Henry, Dornford Yates, Maurice Walsh, De Maupassant, Victor Hugo, Sapper, C.N. Williamson, "Bartimeus" and the crown of her collection- Dickens "The Old Curiosity Shop," and so on… Just call her "Renaissance Woman" - collecting herbal remedies, acting like Universal Helping Hand/Agony Aunt, or escaping to her dear mountains for a bit of exploring, collecting herbs and plants, and trekking.

Check out some of the other JD-Biz Publishing books

Gardening Series on Amazon

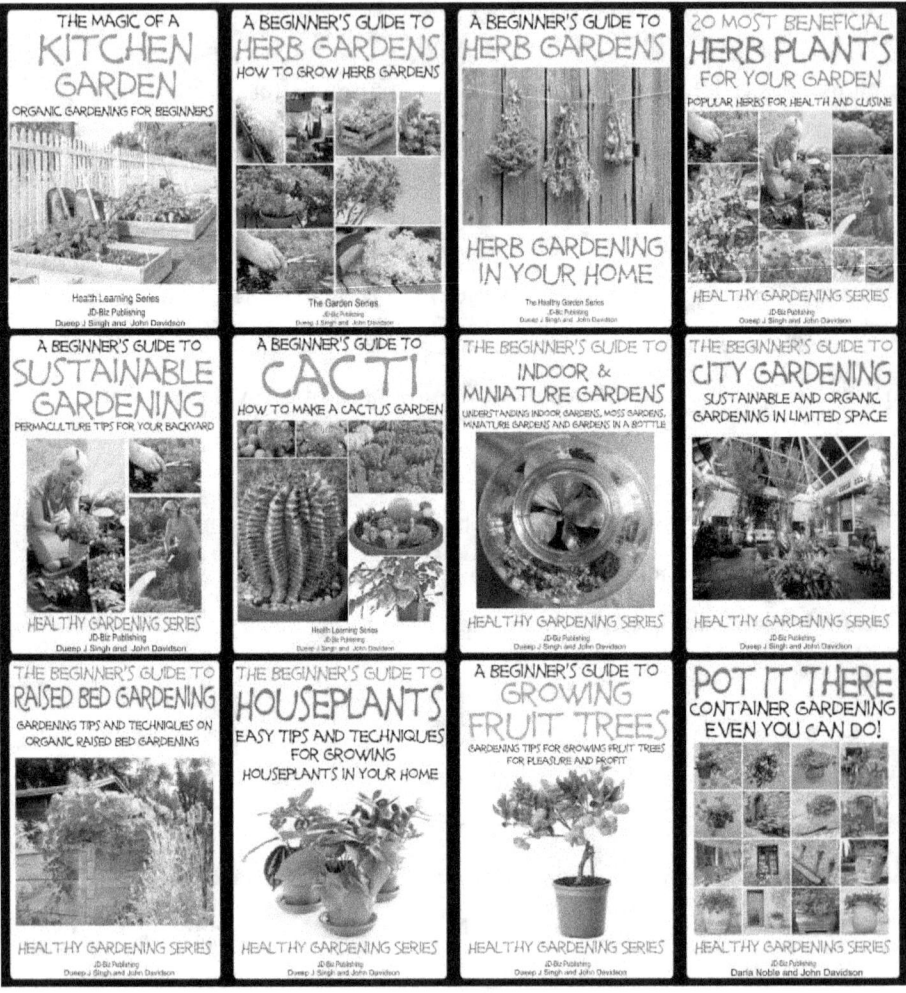

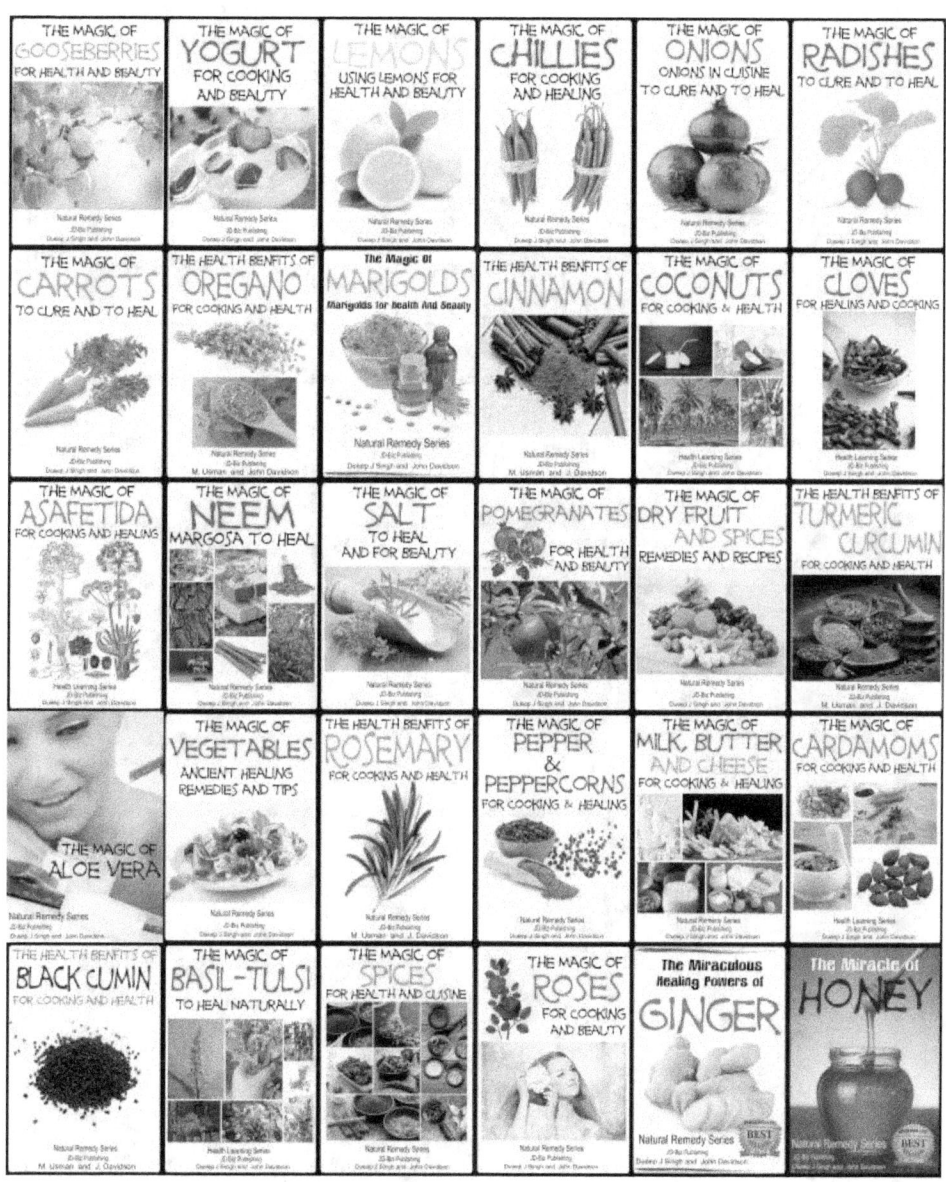

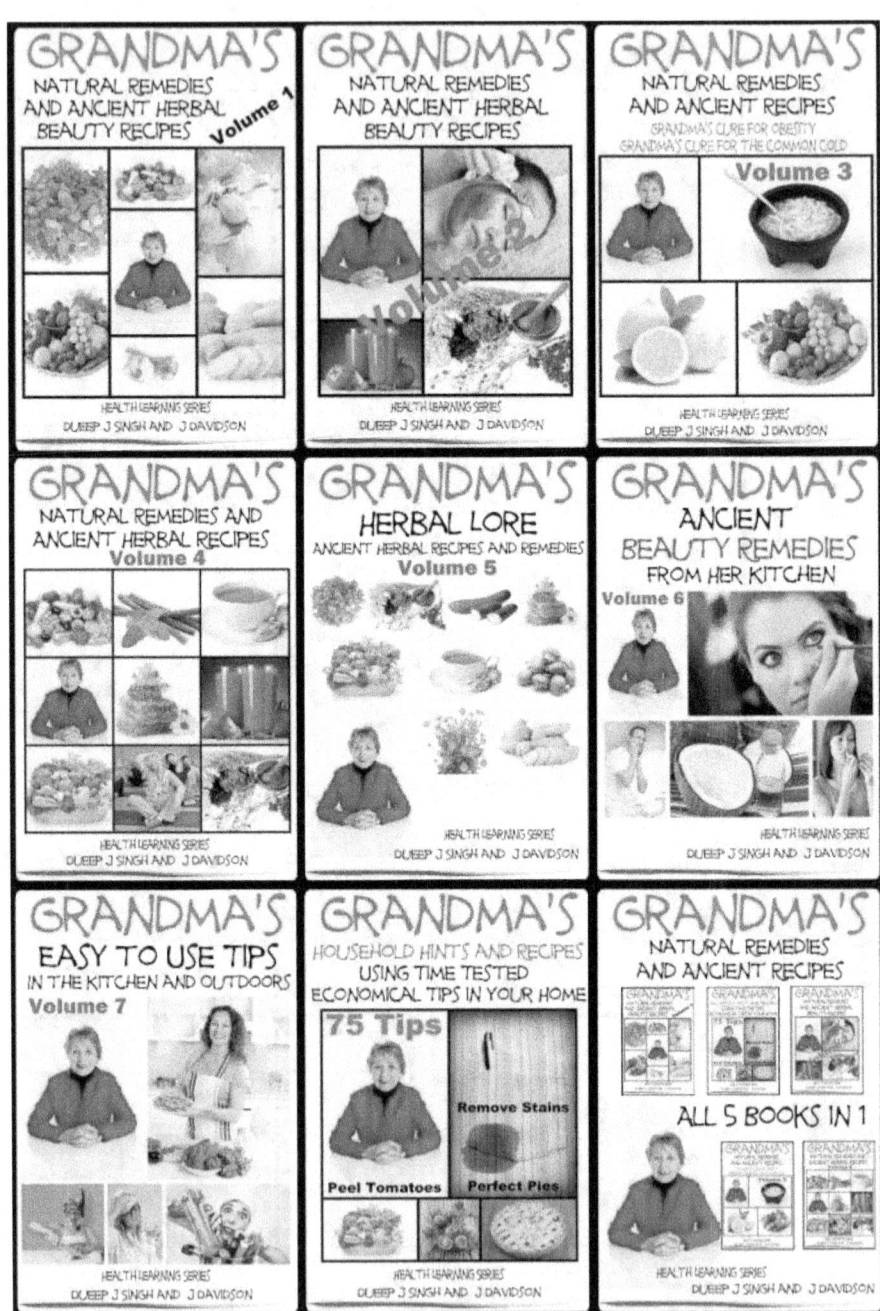

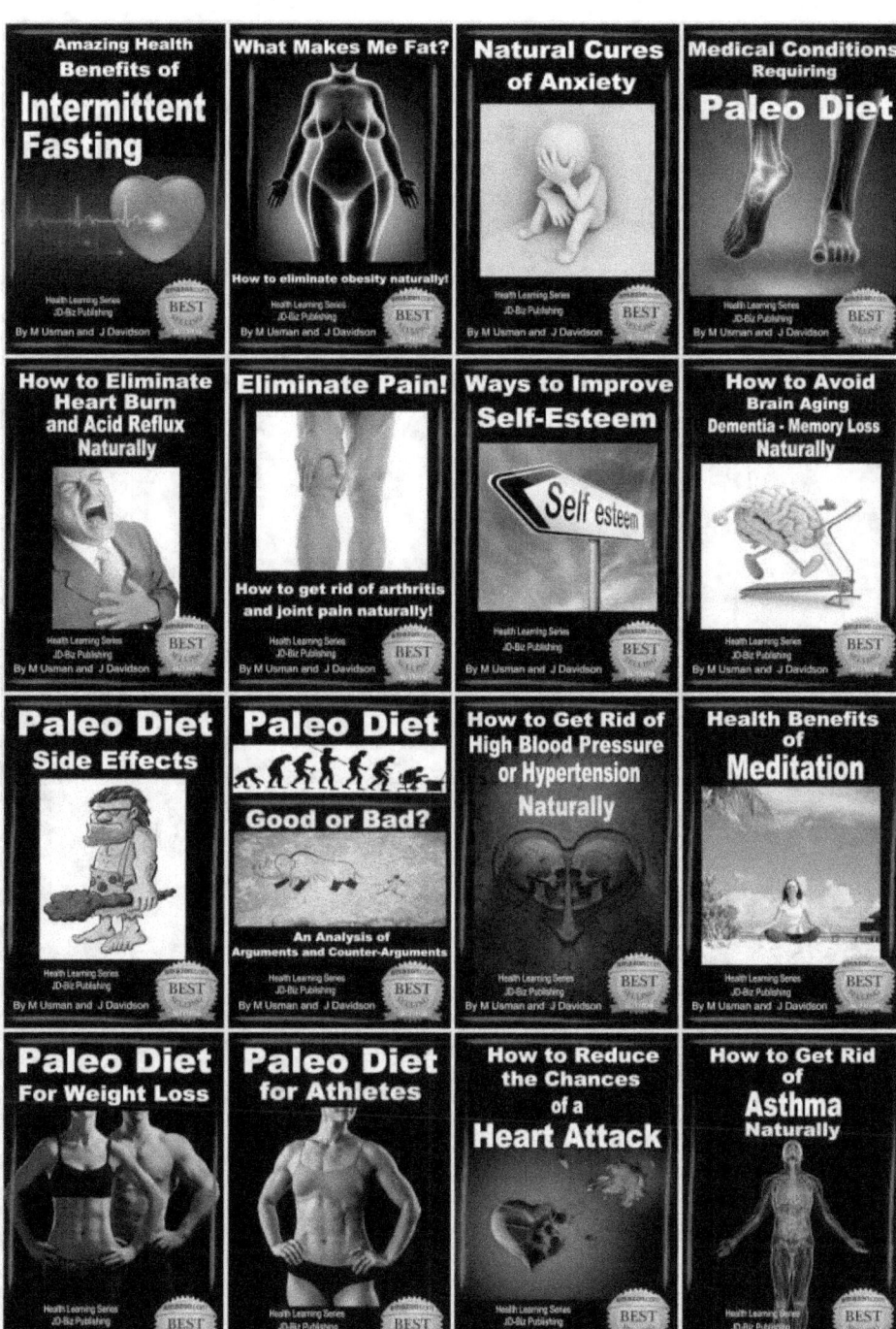

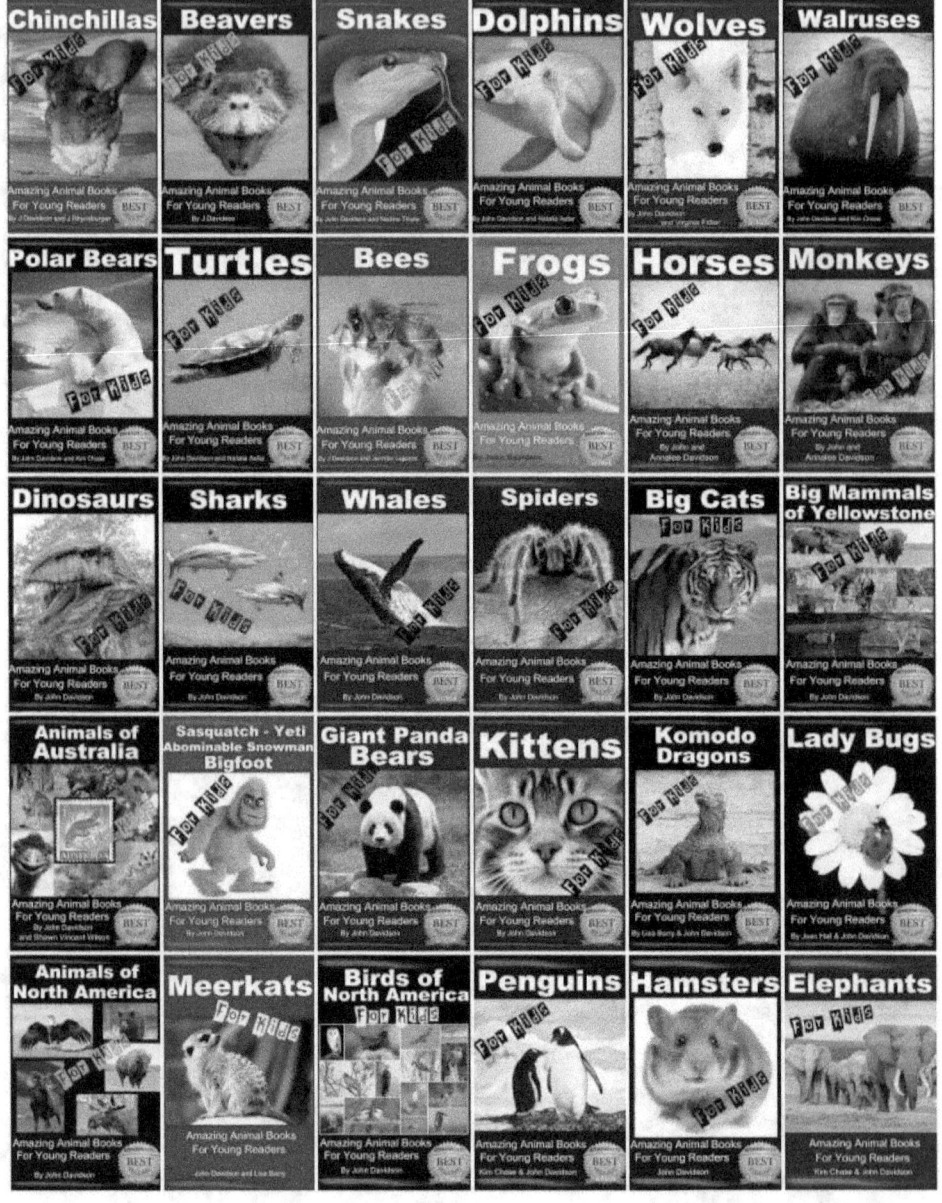

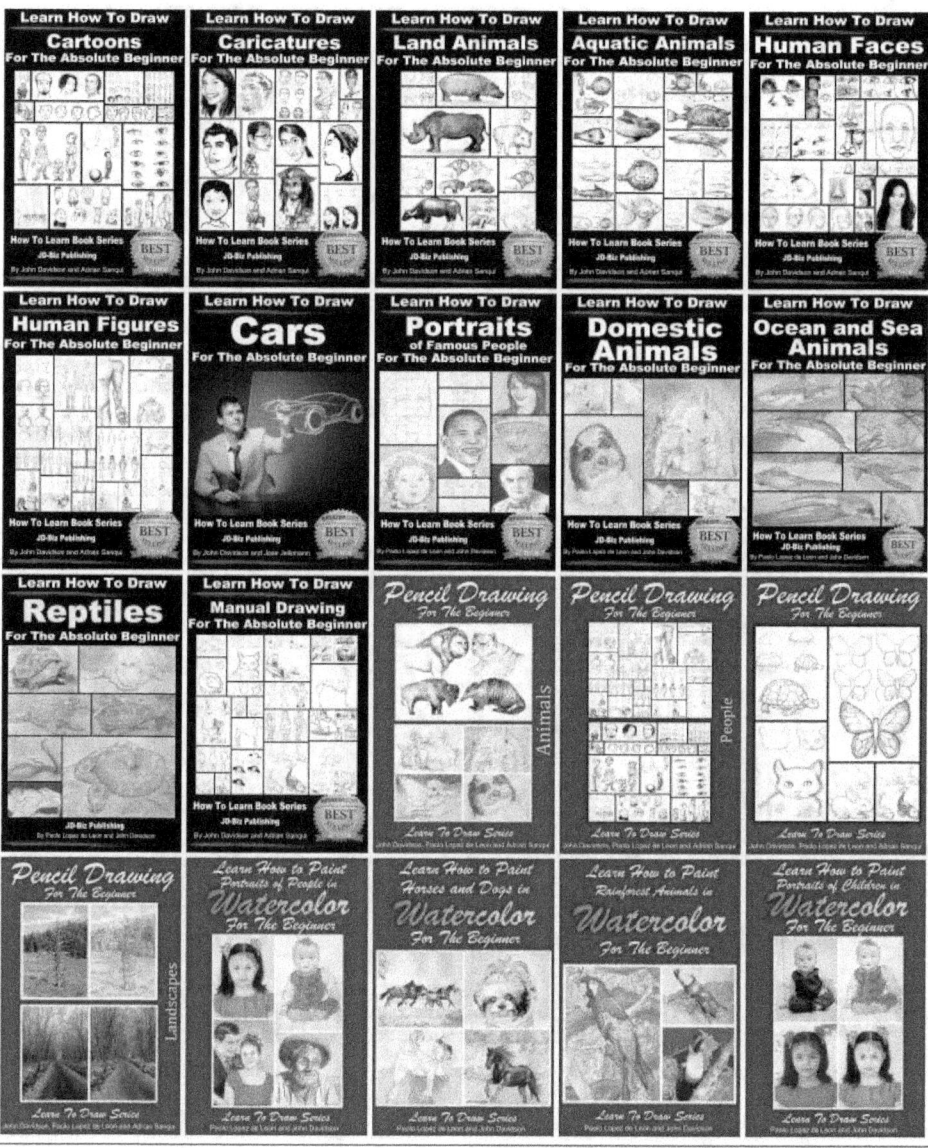

How to Build and Plan Books

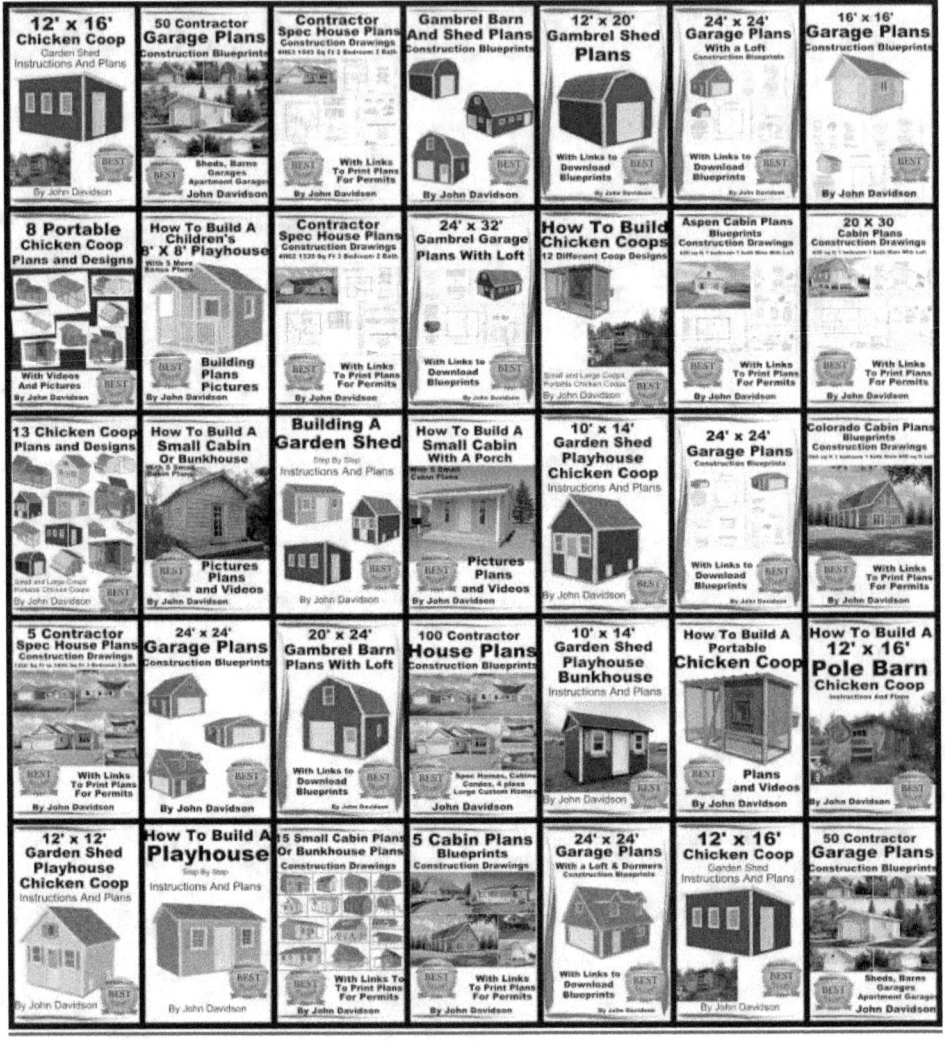

Entrepreneur Book Series

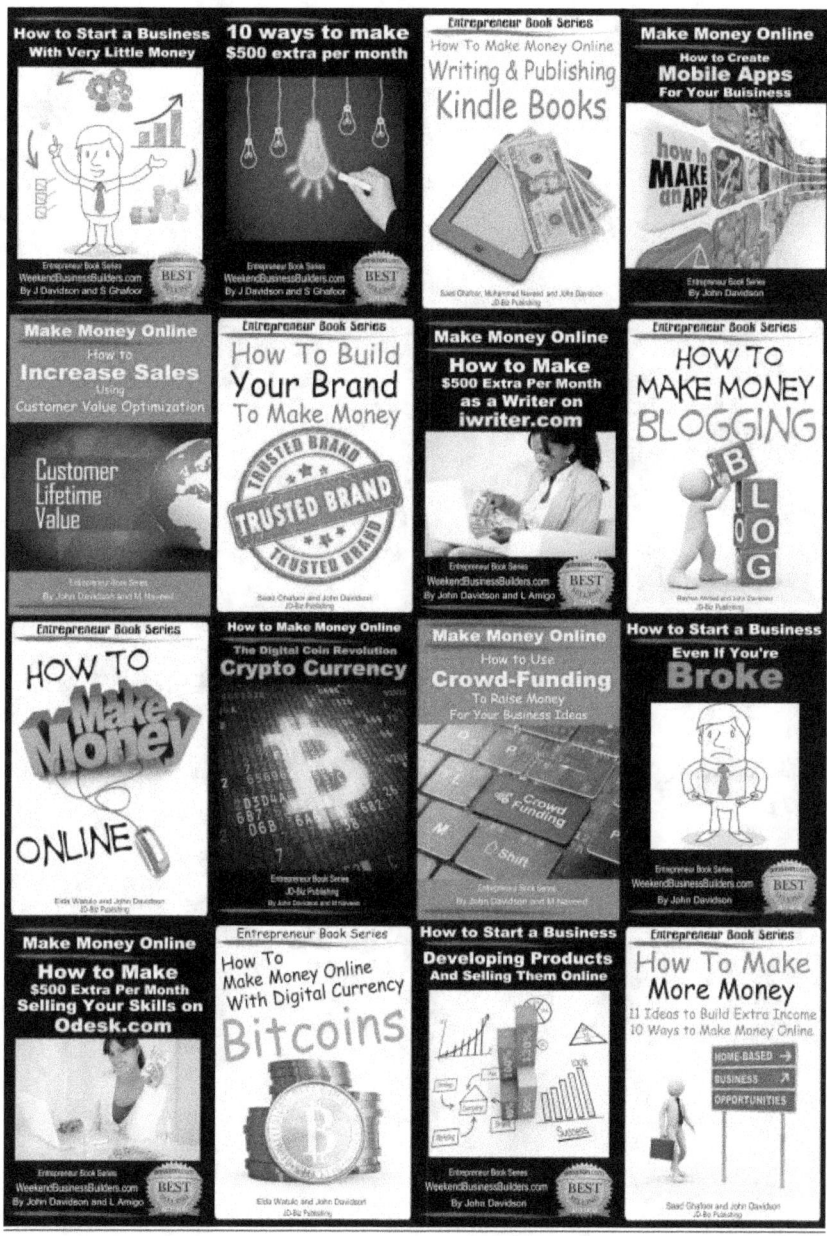

Our books are available at

1. Amazon.com

2. Barnes and Noble

3. Itunes

4. Kobo

5. Smashwords

6. Google Play Books

Download Free Books!

http://MendonCottageBooks.com

Publisher

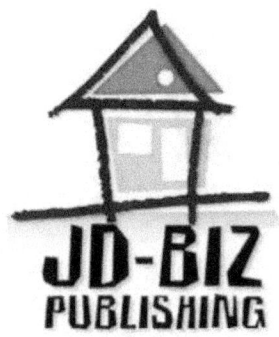

JD-Biz Corp

P O Box 374

Mendon, Utah 84325

http://www.jd-biz.com/

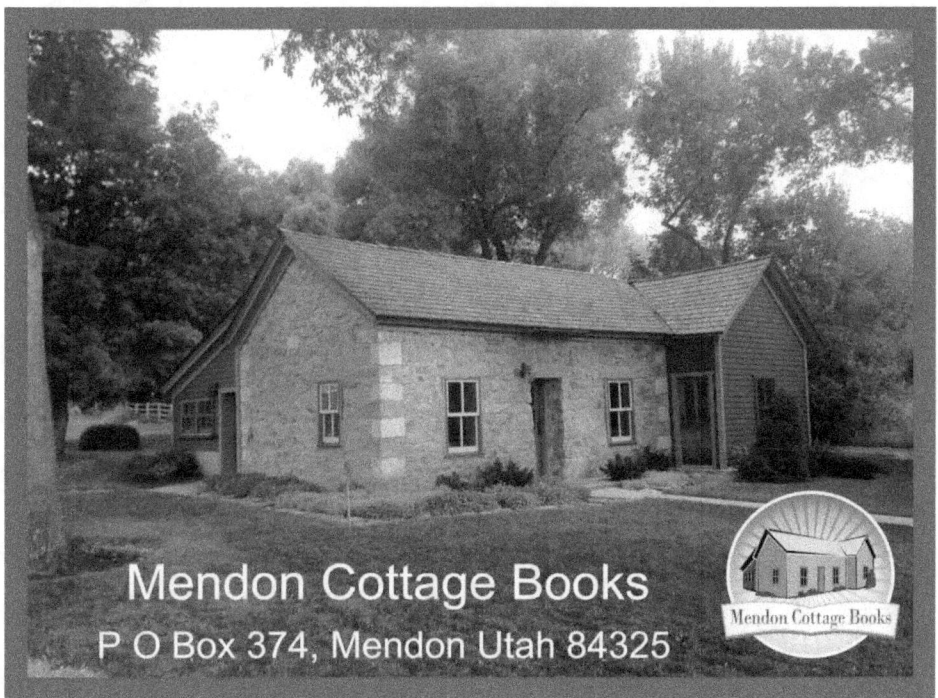

www.ingramcontent.com/pod-product-compliance
Lightning Source LLC
Chambersburg PA
CBHW071126280526
45787CB00003B/1193